This Medical Cannabis Journal Belongs To

_____

Strain

Grower _____ Date _____

Acquired _____ $ _____

| Indica | Hybrid | Sativa |

☐ Flower ☐ Edible ☐ Concentrate

Symptoms Relieved

_____
_____
_____
_____
_____

Sweet · Floral · Spicy · Herbal · Woodsy · Earthy · Sour · Fruity

Notes

_____
_____
_____
_____
_____
_____

Effects	Strength
Peaceful	○ ○ ○ ○ ○
Sleepy	○ ○ ○ ○ ○
Pain Relief	○ ○ ○ ○ ○
Hungry	○ ○ ○ ○ ○
Uplifted	○ ○ ○ ○ ○
Creative	○ ○ ○ ○ ○

Ratings ☆ ☆ ☆ ☆ ☆

Strain

Grower _____ Date _____

Acquired _____ $ _____

| Indica | Hybrid | Sativa |

☐ Flower ☐ Edible ☐ Concentrate

Symptoms Relieved

_____
_____
_____
_____
_____

Sweet / Floral / Spicy / Herbal / Woodsy / Earthy / Sour / Fruity

Notes

_____
_____
_____
_____
_____
_____

Effects	Strength
Peaceful	○ ○ ○ ○ ○
Sleepy	○ ○ ○ ○ ○
Pain Relief	○ ○ ○ ○ ○
Hungry	○ ○ ○ ○ ○
Uplifted	○ ○ ○ ○ ○
Creative	○ ○ ○ ○ ○

Ratings ☆ ☆ ☆ ☆ ☆

Strain

Grower _____ Date _____

Acquired _____ $ _____

| Indica | Hybrid | Sativa |

☐ Flower ☐ Edible ☐ Concentrate

Symptoms Relieved

_____
_____
_____
_____

Sweet / Fruity / Floral / Sour / Spicy / Earthy / Woodsy / Herbal

Notes

_____
_____
_____
_____
_____
_____
_____

Effects	Strength
Peaceful	○ ○ ○ ○ ○
Sleepy	○ ○ ○ ○ ○
Pain Relief	○ ○ ○ ○ ○
Hungry	○ ○ ○ ○ ○
Uplifted	○ ○ ○ ○ ○
Creative	○ ○ ○ ○ ○

Ratings ☆ ☆ ☆ ☆ ☆

Strain

Grower _____ Date _____

Acquired _____ $ _____

| Indica | Hybrid | Sativa |

☐ Flower ☐ Edible ☐ Concentrate

Sweet
Fruity — Floral
Sour — Spicy
Earthy — Herbal
Woodsy

Symptoms Relieved

_____
_____
_____
_____

Notes

_____
_____
_____
_____
_____

Effects	Strength
Peaceful	○ ○ ○ ○ ○
Sleepy	○ ○ ○ ○ ○
Pain Relief	○ ○ ○ ○ ○
Hungry	○ ○ ○ ○ ○
Uplifted	○ ○ ○ ○ ○
Creative	○ ○ ○ ○ ○

Ratings ☆ ☆ ☆ ☆ ☆

Strain

Grower _____ Date _____

Acquired _____ $ _____

Indica   Hybrid   Sativa

☐ Flower   ☐ Edible   ☐ Concentrate

Symptoms Relieved

_____
_____
_____
_____

Sweet • Floral • Spicy • Herbal • Woodsy • Earthy • Sour • Fruity

Notes

_____
_____
_____
_____
_____

Effects	Strength
Peaceful	○ ○ ○ ○ ○
Sleepy	○ ○ ○ ○ ○
Pain Relief	○ ○ ○ ○ ○
Hungry	○ ○ ○ ○ ○
Uplifted	○ ○ ○ ○ ○
Creative	○ ○ ○ ○ ○

Ratings ☆ ☆ ☆ ☆ ☆

Strain

Grower _____ Date _____

Acquired _____ $ _____

| Indica | Hybrid | Sativa |

☐ Flower ☐ Edible ☐ Concentrate

Symptoms Relieved

_____
_____
_____
_____
_____

Sweet · Floral · Spicy · Herbal · Woodsy · Earthy · Sour · Fruity

Notes

_____
_____
_____
_____
_____
_____
_____

Effects	Strength
Peaceful	○ ○ ○ ○ ○
Sleepy	○ ○ ○ ○ ○
Pain Relief	○ ○ ○ ○ ○
Hungry	○ ○ ○ ○ ○
Uplifted	○ ○ ○ ○ ○
Creative	○ ○ ○ ○ ○

Ratings ☆ ☆ ☆ ☆ ☆

Strain

Grower _____ Date _____

Acquired _____ $ _____

| Indica | Hybrid | Sativa |

☐ Flower ☐ Edible ☐ Concentrate

Symptoms Relieved

_____
_____
_____
_____
_____

Sweet / Fruity / Floral / Spicy / Herbal / Woodsy / Earthy / Sour

Notes

_____
_____
_____
_____
_____
_____

Effects	Strength
Peaceful	○ ○ ○ ○ ○
Sleepy	○ ○ ○ ○ ○
Pain Relief	○ ○ ○ ○ ○
Hungry	○ ○ ○ ○ ○
Uplifted	○ ○ ○ ○ ○
Creative	○ ○ ○ ○ ○

Ratings ☆ ☆ ☆ ☆ ☆

Strain

Grower _____ Date _____

Acquired _____ $ _____

| Indica | Hybrid | Sativa |

☐ Flower ☐ Edible ☐ Concentrate

Sweet
Fruity   Floral
Sour   Spicy
Earthy   Herbal
Woodsy

Symptoms Relieved

_____
_____
_____
_____

Notes

_____
_____
_____
_____

Effects	Strength
Peaceful	○ ○ ○ ○ ○
Sleepy	○ ○ ○ ○ ○
Pain Relief	○ ○ ○ ○ ○
Hungry	○ ○ ○ ○ ○
Uplifted	○ ○ ○ ○ ○
Creative	○ ○ ○ ○ ○

Ratings ☆ ☆ ☆ ☆ ☆

Strain

Grower _____ Date _____

Acquired _____ $ _____

| Indica | Hybrid | Sativa |

☐ Flower ☐ Edible ☐ Concentrate

Sweet
Fruity   Floral
Sour   Spicy
Earthy   Herbal
Woodsy

Symptoms Relieved

_____
_____
_____
_____
_____

Notes

_____
_____
_____
_____
_____
_____
_____

Effects **Strength**

Peaceful   ○ ○ ○ ○ ○
Sleepy   ○ ○ ○ ○ ○
Pain Relief ○ ○ ○ ○ ○
Hungry   ○ ○ ○ ○ ○
Uplifted   ○ ○ ○ ○ ○
Creative   ○ ○ ○ ○ ○

Ratings ☆ ☆ ☆ ☆ ☆

Strain

Grower _____   Date _____

Acquired _____ $ _____

| Indica | Hybrid | Sativa |

☐ Flower   ☐ Edible   ☐ Concentrate

Symptoms Relieved

_____
_____
_____
_____
_____

Sweet
Fruity
Floral
Sour
Spicy
Earthy
Herbal
Woodsy

Notes

_____
_____
_____
_____
_____
_____
_____

Effects	Strength
Peaceful	○ ○ ○ ○ ○
Sleepy	○ ○ ○ ○ ○
Pain Relief	○ ○ ○ ○ ○
Hungry	○ ○ ○ ○ ○
Uplifted	○ ○ ○ ○ ○
Creative	○ ○ ○ ○ ○

Ratings ☆ ☆ ☆ ☆ ☆

Strain

Grower _____ Date _____

Acquired _____ $ _____

Indica   Hybrid   Sativa

☐ Flower   ☐ Edible   ☐ Concentrate

Sweet
Fruity   Floral
Sour   Spicy
Earthy   Herbal
Woodsy

Symptoms Relieved

_____
_____
_____
_____

Notes

_____
_____
_____
_____
_____
_____

Effects	Strength
Peaceful	○ ○ ○ ○ ○
Sleepy	○ ○ ○ ○ ○
Pain Relief	○ ○ ○ ○ ○
Hungry	○ ○ ○ ○ ○
Uplifted	○ ○ ○ ○ ○
Creative	○ ○ ○ ○ ○

Ratings ☆ ☆ ☆ ☆ ☆

Strain

Grower _____ Date _____

Acquired _____ $ _____

| Indica | Hybrid | Sativa |

☐ Flower ☐ Edible ☐ Concentrate

Symptoms Relieved

_____
_____
_____
_____
_____

Sweet · Floral · Spicy · Herbal · Woodsy · Earthy · Sour · Fruity

Notes

_____
_____
_____
_____
_____
_____
_____

Effects	Strength
Peaceful	○ ○ ○ ○ ○
Sleepy	○ ○ ○ ○ ○
Pain Relief	○ ○ ○ ○ ○
Hungry	○ ○ ○ ○ ○
Uplifted	○ ○ ○ ○ ○
Creative	○ ○ ○ ○ ○

Ratings ☆ ☆ ☆ ☆ ☆

Strain

Grower _____ Date _____

Acquired _____ $ _____

| Indica | Hybrid | Sativa |

☐ Flower ☐ Edible ☐ Concentrate

Sweet · Fruity · Floral · Sour · Spicy · Earthy · Herbal · Woodsy

Symptoms Relieved

_____
_____
_____
_____

Notes

_____
_____
_____
_____
_____
_____

Effects	Strength
Peaceful	○ ○ ○ ○ ○
Sleepy	○ ○ ○ ○ ○
Pain Relief	○ ○ ○ ○ ○
Hungry	○ ○ ○ ○ ○
Uplifted	○ ○ ○ ○ ○
Creative	○ ○ ○ ○ ○

Ratings ☆ ☆ ☆ ☆ ☆

Strain

Grower _____ Date _____

Acquired _____ $ _____

| Indica | Hybrid | Sativa |

☐ Flower   ☐ Edible   ☐ Concentrate

Sweet
Fruity   Floral
Sour   Spicy
Earthy   Herbal
Woodsy

Symptoms Relieved

_____
_____
_____
_____

Notes

_____
_____
_____
_____
_____

Effects	Strength
Peaceful	○ ○ ○ ○ ○
Sleepy	○ ○ ○ ○ ○
Pain Relief	○ ○ ○ ○ ○
Hungry	○ ○ ○ ○ ○
Uplifted	○ ○ ○ ○ ○
Creative	○ ○ ○ ○ ○

Ratings ☆ ☆ ☆ ☆ ☆

Strain

Grower _____ Date _____

Acquired _____ $ _____

| Indica | Hybrid | Sativa |

☐ Flower ☐ Edible ☐ Concentrate

Sweet · Floral · Spicy · Herbal · Woodsy · Earthy · Sour · Fruity

Symptoms Relieved

_____
_____
_____
_____
_____

Notes

_____
_____
_____
_____
_____

Effects	Strength
Peaceful	○ ○ ○ ○ ○
Sleepy	○ ○ ○ ○ ○
Pain Relief	○ ○ ○ ○ ○
Hungry	○ ○ ○ ○ ○
Uplifted	○ ○ ○ ○ ○
Creative	○ ○ ○ ○ ○

Ratings ☆ ☆ ☆ ☆ ☆

Strain

Grower _____ Date _____

Acquired _____ $ _____

| Indica | Hybrid | Sativa |

☐ Flower ☐ Edible ☐ Concentrate

Symptoms Relieved

_____
_____
_____
_____

Sweet
Fruity   Floral
Sour   Spicy
Earthy   Herbal
Woodsy

Notes

_____
_____
_____
_____
_____
_____
_____

Effects	**Strength**
Peaceful	○ ○ ○ ○ ○
Sleepy	○ ○ ○ ○ ○
Pain Relief	○ ○ ○ ○ ○
Hungry	○ ○ ○ ○ ○
Uplifted	○ ○ ○ ○ ○
Creative	○ ○ ○ ○ ○

Ratings ☆ ☆ ☆ ☆ ☆

Strain

Grower _____ Date _____

Acquired _____ $ _____

| Indica | Hybrid | Sativa |

☐ Flower   ☐ Edible   ☐ Concentrate

Sweet · Fruity · Floral · Sour · Spicy · Earthy · Woodsy · Herbal

Symptoms Relieved

_____
_____
_____
_____

Notes

_____
_____
_____
_____
_____
_____

Effects	Strength
Peaceful	○ ○ ○ ○ ○
Sleepy	○ ○ ○ ○ ○
Pain Relief	○ ○ ○ ○ ○
Hungry	○ ○ ○ ○ ○
Uplifted	○ ○ ○ ○ ○
Creative	○ ○ ○ ○ ○

Ratings ☆ ☆ ☆ ☆ ☆

Strain

Grower _____ Date _____

Acquired _____ $ _____

| Indica | Hybrid | Sativa |

☐ Flower   ☐ Edible   ☐ Concentrate

Symptoms Relieved

_____
_____
_____
_____
_____

Sweet · Floral · Spicy · Herbal · Woodsy · Earthy · Sour · Fruity

Notes

_____
_____
_____
_____
_____
_____
_____

Effects	Strength
Peaceful	○ ○ ○ ○ ○
Sleepy	○ ○ ○ ○ ○
Pain Relief	○ ○ ○ ○ ○
Hungry	○ ○ ○ ○ ○
Uplifted	○ ○ ○ ○ ○
Creative	○ ○ ○ ○ ○

Ratings ☆ ☆ ☆ ☆ ☆

Strain

Grower _____ Date _____

Acquired _____ $ _____

| Indica   Hybrid   Sativa |

☐ Flower   ☐ Edible   ☐ Concentrate

Symptoms Relieved

_____
_____
_____
_____
_____

Sweet · Floral · Spicy · Herbal · Woodsy · Earthy · Sour · Fruity

Notes

_____
_____
_____
_____
_____
_____
_____

Effects	Strength
Peaceful	○ ○ ○ ○ ○
Sleepy	○ ○ ○ ○ ○
Pain Relief	○ ○ ○ ○ ○
Hungry	○ ○ ○ ○ ○
Uplifted	○ ○ ○ ○ ○
Creative	○ ○ ○ ○ ○

Ratings ☆ ☆ ☆ ☆ ☆

Strain

Grower _____ Date _____

Acquired _____ $ _____

| Indica | Hybrid | Sativa |

☐ Flower ☐ Edible ☐ Concentrate

Symptoms Relieved

_____
_____
_____
_____
_____

Sweet · Floral · Spicy · Herbal · Woodsy · Earthy · Sour · Fruity

Notes

_____
_____
_____
_____
_____
_____
_____

Effects	Strength
Peaceful	○ ○ ○ ○ ○
Sleepy	○ ○ ○ ○ ○
Pain Relief	○ ○ ○ ○ ○
Hungry	○ ○ ○ ○ ○
Uplifted	○ ○ ○ ○ ○
Creative	○ ○ ○ ○ ○

Ratings ☆ ☆ ☆ ☆ ☆

Strain

Grower _____ Date _____

Acquired _____ $ _____

| Indica | Hybrid | Sativa |

☐ Flower   ☐ Edible   ☐ Concentrate

Sweet
Fruity   Floral
Sour   Spicy
Earthy   Herbal
Woodsy

Symptoms Relieved
_____
_____
_____
_____
_____

Notes
_____
_____
_____
_____
_____
_____

Effects	Strength
Peaceful	○ ○ ○ ○ ○
Sleepy	○ ○ ○ ○ ○
Pain Relief	○ ○ ○ ○ ○
Hungry	○ ○ ○ ○ ○
Uplifted	○ ○ ○ ○ ○
Creative	○ ○ ○ ○ ○

Ratings ☆ ☆ ☆ ☆ ☆

Strain

Grower _____ Date _____

Acquired _____ $ _____

| Indica | Hybrid | Sativa |

☐ Flower ☐ Edible ☐ Concentrate

Sweet · Floral · Spicy · Herbal · Woodsy · Earthy · Sour · Fruity

Symptoms Relieved

_____
_____
_____
_____
_____

Notes

_____
_____
_____
_____
_____
_____

Effects	Strength
Peaceful	○ ○ ○ ○ ○
Sleepy	○ ○ ○ ○ ○
Pain Relief	○ ○ ○ ○ ○
Hungry	○ ○ ○ ○ ○
Uplifted	○ ○ ○ ○ ○
Creative	○ ○ ○ ○ ○

Ratings ☆ ☆ ☆ ☆ ☆

Strain

Grower _____ Date _____

Acquired _____ $ _____

Indica   Hybrid   Sativa

☐ Flower   ☐ Edible   ☐ Concentrate

Symptoms Relieved

_____
_____
_____
_____

Sweet
Fruity   Floral
Sour   Spicy
Earthy   Herbal
Woodsy

Notes

_____
_____
_____
_____
_____
_____
_____

Effects	Strength
Peaceful	○ ○ ○ ○ ○
Sleepy	○ ○ ○ ○ ○
Pain Relief	○ ○ ○ ○ ○
Hungry	○ ○ ○ ○ ○
Uplifted	○ ○ ○ ○ ○
Creative	○ ○ ○ ○ ○

Ratings ☆ ☆ ☆ ☆ ☆

Strain

Grower _____ Date _____

Acquired _____ $ _____

Indica	Hybrid	Sativa

☐ Flower ☐ Edible ☐ Concentrate

Symptoms Relieved

_____
_____
_____
_____

Sweet · Floral · Spicy · Herbal · Woodsy · Earthy · Sour · Fruity

Notes

_____
_____
_____
_____
_____

Effects	Strength
Peaceful	○ ○ ○ ○ ○
Sleepy	○ ○ ○ ○ ○
Pain Relief	○ ○ ○ ○ ○
Hungry	○ ○ ○ ○ ○
Uplifted	○ ○ ○ ○ ○
Creative	○ ○ ○ ○ ○

Ratings ☆ ☆ ☆ ☆ ☆

Strain

Grower _____ Date _____

Acquired _____ $ _____

Indica   Hybrid   Sativa

☐ Flower ☐ Edible ☐ Concentrate

Symptoms Relieved

_____
_____
_____
_____
_____

Sweet
Fruity   Floral
Sour   Spicy
Earthy   Herbal
Woodsy

Notes

_____
_____
_____
_____
_____
_____
_____

Effects	Strength
Peaceful	○ ○ ○ ○ ○
Sleepy	○ ○ ○ ○ ○
Pain Relief	○ ○ ○ ○ ○
Hungry	○ ○ ○ ○ ○
Uplifted	○ ○ ○ ○ ○
Creative	○ ○ ○ ○ ○

Ratings ☆ ☆ ☆ ☆ ☆

Strain

Grower _____ Date _____

Acquired _____ $ _____

| Indica | Hybrid | Sativa |

☐ Flower ☐ Edible ☐ Concentrate

Symptoms Relieved

_____
_____
_____
_____

Sweet · Fruity · Floral · Sour · Spicy · Earthy · Woodsy · Herbal

Notes

_____
_____
_____
_____
_____

Effects	Strength
Peaceful	○ ○ ○ ○ ○
Sleepy	○ ○ ○ ○ ○
Pain Relief	○ ○ ○ ○ ○
Hungry	○ ○ ○ ○ ○
Uplifted	○ ○ ○ ○ ○
Creative	○ ○ ○ ○ ○

Ratings ☆ ☆ ☆ ☆ ☆

Strain

Grower _____ Date _____

Acquired _____ $ _____

| Indica | Hybrid | Sativa |

☐ Flower   ☐ Edible   ☐ Concentrate

Symptoms Relieved

_____
_____
_____
_____
_____

Sweet · Fruity · Floral · Sour · Spicy · Earthy · Woodsy · Herbal

Notes

_____
_____
_____
_____
_____
_____

Effects	Strength
Peaceful	○ ○ ○ ○ ○
Sleepy	○ ○ ○ ○ ○
Pain Relief	○ ○ ○ ○ ○
Hungry	○ ○ ○ ○ ○
Uplifted	○ ○ ○ ○ ○
Creative	○ ○ ○ ○ ○

Ratings ☆ ☆ ☆ ☆ ☆

Strain

Grower _____ Date _____

Acquired _____ $ _____

| Indica | Hybrid | Sativa |

☐ Flower ☐ Edible ☐ Concentrate

Sweet · Floral · Spicy · Herbal · Woodsy · Earthy · Sour · Fruity

Symptoms Relieved

_____
_____
_____
_____

Notes

_____
_____
_____
_____
_____
_____

Effects	Strength
Peaceful	○ ○ ○ ○ ○
Sleepy	○ ○ ○ ○ ○
Pain Relief	○ ○ ○ ○ ○
Hungry	○ ○ ○ ○ ○
Uplifted	○ ○ ○ ○ ○
Creative	○ ○ ○ ○ ○

Ratings ☆ ☆ ☆ ☆ ☆

Strain

Grower _____ Date _____

Acquired _____ $ _____

| Indica | Hybrid | Sativa |

☐ Flower   ☐ Edible   ☐ Concentrate

Symptoms Relieved

_____
_____
_____
_____

Sweet · Floral · Spicy · Herbal · Woodsy · Earthy · Sour · Fruity

Notes

_____
_____
_____
_____
_____
_____
_____

Effects	Strength
Peaceful	○ ○ ○ ○ ○
Sleepy	○ ○ ○ ○ ○
Pain Relief	○ ○ ○ ○ ○
Hungry	○ ○ ○ ○ ○
Uplifted	○ ○ ○ ○ ○
Creative	○ ○ ○ ○ ○

Ratings ☆ ☆ ☆ ☆ ☆

Strain

Grower _____ Date _____

Acquired _____ $ _____

| Indica | Hybrid | Sativa |

☐ Flower ☐ Edible ☐ Concentrate

Symptoms Relieved

_____
_____
_____
_____

Sweet / Floral / Spicy / Herbal / Woodsy / Earthy / Sour / Fruity

Notes

_____
_____
_____
_____
_____
_____

Effects	Strength
Peaceful	○ ○ ○ ○ ○
Sleepy	○ ○ ○ ○ ○
Pain Relief	○ ○ ○ ○ ○
Hungry	○ ○ ○ ○ ○
Uplifted	○ ○ ○ ○ ○
Creative	○ ○ ○ ○ ○

Ratings ☆ ☆ ☆ ☆ ☆

Strain

Grower _____ Date _____

Acquired _____ $ _____

| Indica | Hybrid | Sativa |

☐ Flower   ☐ Edible   ☐ Concentrate

Symptoms Relieved

_____
_____
_____
_____

Sweet
Fruity   Floral
Sour   Spicy
Earthy   Herbal
Woodsy

Notes

_____
_____
_____
_____
_____
_____

Effects	Strength
Peaceful	○ ○ ○ ○ ○
Sleepy	○ ○ ○ ○ ○
Pain Relief	○ ○ ○ ○ ○
Hungry	○ ○ ○ ○ ○
Uplifted	○ ○ ○ ○ ○
Creative	○ ○ ○ ○ ○

Ratings ☆ ☆ ☆ ☆ ☆

Strain

Grower: _____ Date: _____

Acquired: _____ $ _____

| Indica | Hybrid | Sativa |

☐ Flower ☐ Edible ☐ Concentrate

Sweet · Fruity · Floral · Sour · Spicy · Earthy · Woodsy · Herbal

Symptoms Relieved

_____
_____
_____
_____
_____

Notes

_____
_____
_____
_____
_____
_____

Effects	Strength
Peaceful	○ ○ ○ ○ ○
Sleepy	○ ○ ○ ○ ○
Pain Relief	○ ○ ○ ○ ○
Hungry	○ ○ ○ ○ ○
Uplifted	○ ○ ○ ○ ○
Creative	○ ○ ○ ○ ○

Ratings ☆ ☆ ☆ ☆ ☆

Strain

Grower _____ Date _____

Acquired _____ $ _____

| Indica | Hybrid | Sativa |

☐ Flower ☐ Edible ☐ Concentrate

Symptoms Relieved

_____
_____
_____
_____

Sweet / Floral / Spicy / Herbal / Woodsy / Earthy / Sour / Fruity

Notes

_____
_____
_____
_____
_____
_____
_____

Effects	Strength
Peaceful	○ ○ ○ ○ ○
Sleepy	○ ○ ○ ○ ○
Pain Relief	○ ○ ○ ○ ○
Hungry	○ ○ ○ ○ ○
Uplifted	○ ○ ○ ○ ○
Creative	○ ○ ○ ○ ○

Ratings ☆ ☆ ☆ ☆ ☆

Strain

Grower _____ Date _____

Acquired _____ $ _____

| Indica | Hybrid | Sativa |

☐ Flower ☐ Edible ☐ Concentrate

Sweet
Fruity   Floral

Sour   Spicy

Earthy   Herbal
Woodsy

Symptoms Relieved
_____
_____
_____
_____

Notes
_____
_____
_____
_____
_____
_____

Effects	Strength
Peaceful	○ ○ ○ ○ ○
Sleepy	○ ○ ○ ○ ○
Pain Relief	○ ○ ○ ○ ○
Hungry	○ ○ ○ ○ ○
Uplifted	○ ○ ○ ○ ○
Creative	○ ○ ○ ○ ○

Ratings ☆ ☆ ☆ ☆ ☆

Strain

Grower _____   Date _____

Acquired _____ $ _____

Indica   Hybrid   Sativa

☐ Flower   ☐ Edible   ☐ Concentrate

Symptoms Relieved

_____
_____
_____
_____

Sweet
Fruity   Floral
Sour   Spicy
Earthy   Herbal
Woodsy

Notes

_____
_____
_____
_____
_____
_____

Effects	Strength
Peaceful	○ ○ ○ ○ ○
Sleepy	○ ○ ○ ○ ○
Pain Relief	○ ○ ○ ○ ○
Hungry	○ ○ ○ ○ ○
Uplifted	○ ○ ○ ○ ○
Creative	○ ○ ○ ○ ○

Ratings ☆ ☆ ☆ ☆

Strain

Grower _____ Date _____

Acquired _____ $ _____

Indica	Hybrid	Sativa

☐ Flower ☐ Edible ☐ Concentrate

Symptoms Relieved

_____
_____
_____
_____
_____

Sweet · Floral · Spicy · Herbal · Woodsy · Earthy · Sour · Fruity

Notes

_____
_____
_____
_____
_____
_____

Effects	Strength
Peaceful	○ ○ ○ ○ ○
Sleepy	○ ○ ○ ○ ○
Pain Relief	○ ○ ○ ○ ○
Hungry	○ ○ ○ ○ ○
Uplifted	○ ○ ○ ○ ○
Creative	○ ○ ○ ○ ○

Ratings ☆ ☆ ☆ ☆ ☆

Strain

Grower _____   Date _____

Acquired _____ $ _____

| Indica | Hybrid | Sativa |

☐ Flower   ☐ Edible   ☐ Concentrate

Symptoms Relieved

_____
_____
_____
_____

Sweet · Fruity · Floral · Sour · Spicy · Earthy · Herbal · Woodsy

Notes

_____
_____
_____
_____
_____
_____

Effects	Strength
Peaceful	○ ○ ○ ○ ○
Sleepy	○ ○ ○ ○ ○
Pain Relief	○ ○ ○ ○ ○
Hungry	○ ○ ○ ○ ○
Uplifted	○ ○ ○ ○ ○
Creative	○ ○ ○ ○ ○

Ratings ☆ ☆ ☆ ☆ ☆

Strain

Grower _____ Date _____

Acquired _____ $ _____

| Indica | Hybrid | Sativa |

☐ Flower ☐ Edible ☐ Concentrate

Flavor wheel: Sweet, Floral, Spicy, Herbal, Woodsy, Earthy, Sour, Fruity

Symptoms Relieved

_____
_____
_____
_____

Notes

_____
_____
_____
_____
_____
_____

Effects	Strength
Peaceful	○ ○ ○ ○ ○
Sleepy	○ ○ ○ ○ ○
Pain Relief	○ ○ ○ ○ ○
Hungry	○ ○ ○ ○ ○
Uplifted	○ ○ ○ ○ ○
Creative	○ ○ ○ ○ ○

Ratings ☆ ☆ ☆ ☆ ☆

Strain

Grower _____ Date _____

Acquired _____ $ _____

| Indica   Hybrid   Sativa |

☐ Flower   ☐ Edible   ☐ Concentrate

Symptoms Relieved

_____
_____
_____
_____
_____

Sweet / Fruity / Floral / Sour / Spicy / Earthy / Woodsy / Herbal

Notes

_____
_____
_____
_____
_____
_____
_____

Effects	Strength
Peaceful	○ ○ ○ ○ ○
Sleepy	○ ○ ○ ○ ○
Pain Relief	○ ○ ○ ○ ○
Hungry	○ ○ ○ ○ ○
Uplifted	○ ○ ○ ○ ○
Creative	○ ○ ○ ○ ○

Ratings ☆ ☆ ☆ ☆ ☆

Strain

Grower _____ Date _____

Acquired _____ $ _____

Indica	Hybrid	Sativa

☐ Flower ☐ Edible ☐ Concentrate

Symptoms Relieved

_____
_____
_____
_____
_____

Sweet · Floral · Spicy · Herbal · Woodsy · Earthy · Sour · Fruity

Notes

_____
_____
_____
_____
_____
_____
_____

Effects	Strength
Peaceful	○ ○ ○ ○ ○
Sleepy	○ ○ ○ ○ ○
Pain Relief	○ ○ ○ ○ ○
Hungry	○ ○ ○ ○ ○
Uplifted	○ ○ ○ ○ ○
Creative	○ ○ ○ ○ ○

Ratings ☆ ☆ ☆ ☆ ☆

Strain

Grower _____ Date _____

Acquired _____ $ _____

Indica   Hybrid   Sativa

☐ Flower   ☐ Edible   ☐ Concentrate

Symptoms Relieved

_____
_____
_____
_____

Sweet
Fruity   Floral
Sour   Spicy
Earthy   Herbal
Woodsy

Notes

_____
_____
_____
_____
_____
_____

Effects	Strength
Peaceful	○ ○ ○ ○ ○
Sleepy	○ ○ ○ ○ ○
Pain Relief	○ ○ ○ ○ ○
Hungry	○ ○ ○ ○ ○
Uplifted	○ ○ ○ ○ ○
Creative	○ ○ ○ ○ ○

Ratings ☆ ☆ ☆ ☆ ☆

Strain

Grower: _____ Date: _____

Acquired: _____ $ _____

| Indica | Hybrid | Sativa |

☐ Flower ☐ Edible ☐ Concentrate

Symptoms Relieved

_____
_____
_____
_____

Aroma wheel: Sweet, Floral, Spicy, Herbal, Woodsy, Earthy, Sour, Fruity

Notes

_____
_____
_____
_____
_____
_____
_____

Effects	Strength
Peaceful	○ ○ ○ ○ ○
Sleepy	○ ○ ○ ○ ○
Pain Relief	○ ○ ○ ○ ○
Hungry	○ ○ ○ ○ ○
Uplifted	○ ○ ○ ○ ○
Creative	○ ○ ○ ○ ○

Ratings ☆ ☆ ☆ ☆ ☆

Strain

Grower _____ Date _____

Acquired _____ $ _____

| Indica | Hybrid | Sativa |

☐ Flower   ☐ Edible   ☐ Concentrate

Symptoms Relieved

_____
_____
_____
_____

Sweet / Fruity / Floral / Sour / Spicy / Earthy / Herbal / Woodsy

Notes

_____
_____
_____
_____
_____
_____
_____

Effects	**Strength**
Peaceful	○ ○ ○ ○ ○
Sleepy	○ ○ ○ ○ ○
Pain Relief	○ ○ ○ ○ ○
Hungry	○ ○ ○ ○ ○
Uplifted	○ ○ ○ ○ ○
Creative	○ ○ ○ ○ ○

Ratings ☆ ☆ ☆ ☆ ☆

Strain

Grower _____ Date _____

Acquired _____ $ _____

| Indica | Hybrid | Sativa |

☐ Flower   ☐ Edible   ☐ Concentrate

Symptoms Relieved

_____
_____
_____
_____
_____

Sweet · Fruity · Floral · Sour · Spicy · Earthy · Woodsy · Herbal

Notes

_____
_____
_____
_____
_____
_____

Effects	Strength
Peaceful	○ ○ ○ ○ ○
Sleepy	○ ○ ○ ○ ○
Pain Relief	○ ○ ○ ○ ○
Hungry	○ ○ ○ ○ ○
Uplifted	○ ○ ○ ○ ○
Creative	○ ○ ○ ○ ○

Ratings ☆ ☆ ☆ ☆ ☆

Strain

Grower _____   Date _____

Acquired _____ $ _____

| Indica | Hybrid | Sativa |

☐ Flower   ☐ Edible   ☐ Concentrate

Symptoms Relieved

_____
_____
_____
_____
_____

Sweet / Fruity / Floral / Sour / Spicy / Earthy / Woodsy / Herbal

Notes

_____
_____
_____
_____
_____
_____
_____

Effects	Strength
Peaceful	○ ○ ○ ○ ○
Sleepy	○ ○ ○ ○ ○
Pain Relief	○ ○ ○ ○ ○
Hungry	○ ○ ○ ○ ○
Uplifted	○ ○ ○ ○ ○
Creative	○ ○ ○ ○ ○

Ratings ☆ ☆ ☆ ☆ ☆

Strain

Grower _____ Date _____

Acquired _____ $ _____

| Indica | Hybrid | Sativa |

☐ Flower ☐ Edible ☐ Concentrate

Symptoms Relieved

_____
_____
_____
_____
_____

Sweet · Fruity · Floral · Sour · Spicy · Earthy · Woodsy · Herbal

Notes

_____
_____
_____
_____
_____
_____
_____

Effects	Strength
Peaceful	○ ○ ○ ○ ○
Sleepy	○ ○ ○ ○ ○
Pain Relief	○ ○ ○ ○ ○
Hungry	○ ○ ○ ○ ○
Uplifted	○ ○ ○ ○ ○
Creative	○ ○ ○ ○ ○

Ratings ☆ ☆ ☆ ☆ ☆

Strain

Grower _____ Date _____

Acquired _____ $ _____

| Indica | Hybrid | Sativa |

☐ Flower ☐ Edible ☐ Concentrate

Sweet
Fruity — Floral
Sour — Spicy
Earthy — Herbal
Woodsy

Symptoms Relieved

_____
_____
_____
_____

Notes

_____
_____
_____
_____
_____
_____

Effects	Strength
Peaceful	○ ○ ○ ○ ○
Sleepy	○ ○ ○ ○ ○
Pain Relief	○ ○ ○ ○ ○
Hungry	○ ○ ○ ○ ○
Uplifted	○ ○ ○ ○ ○
Creative	○ ○ ○ ○ ○

Ratings ☆ ☆ ☆ ☆ ☆

Strain

Grower: _____ Date: _____

Acquired: _____ $ _____

| Indica | Hybrid | Sativa |

☐ Flower ☐ Edible ☐ Concentrate

Symptoms Relieved

_____
_____
_____
_____
_____

Flavor wheel: Sweet, Floral, Spicy, Herbal, Woodsy, Earthy, Sour, Fruity

Notes

_____
_____
_____
_____
_____
_____
_____

Effects	Strength
Peaceful	○ ○ ○ ○ ○
Sleepy	○ ○ ○ ○ ○
Pain Relief	○ ○ ○ ○ ○
Hungry	○ ○ ○ ○ ○
Uplifted	○ ○ ○ ○ ○
Creative	○ ○ ○ ○ ○

Ratings ☆ ☆ ☆ ☆ ☆

Strain

Grower _____ Date _____

Acquired _____ $ _____

| Indica | Hybrid | Sativa |

☐ Flower ☐ Edible ☐ Concentrate

Symptoms Relieved

_____
_____
_____
_____

Sweet / Fruity / Floral / Sour / Spicy / Earthy / Woodsy / Herbal

Notes

_____
_____
_____
_____
_____
_____

Effects	Strength
Peaceful	○ ○ ○ ○ ○
Sleepy	○ ○ ○ ○ ○
Pain Relief	○ ○ ○ ○ ○
Hungry	○ ○ ○ ○ ○
Uplifted	○ ○ ○ ○ ○
Creative	○ ○ ○ ○ ○

Ratings ☆ ☆ ☆ ☆ ☆

Strain

Grower _____ Date _____

Acquired _____ $ _____

| Indica | Hybrid | Sativa |

☐ Flower   ☐ Edible   ☐ Concentrate

Symptoms Relieved

_____
_____
_____
_____
_____

Flavor wheel: Sweet, Floral, Spicy, Herbal, Woodsy, Earthy, Sour, Fruity

Notes

_____
_____
_____
_____
_____
_____

Effects	Strength
Peaceful	○ ○ ○ ○ ○
Sleepy	○ ○ ○ ○ ○
Pain Relief	○ ○ ○ ○ ○
Hungry	○ ○ ○ ○ ○
Uplifted	○ ○ ○ ○ ○
Creative	○ ○ ○ ○ ○

Ratings ☆ ☆ ☆ ☆ ☆

Strain

Grower _____ Date _____

Acquired _____ $ _____

| Indica | Hybrid | Sativa |

☐ Flower ☐ Edible ☐ Concentrate

Sweet
Fruity   Floral
Sour   Spicy
Earthy   Herbal
Woodsy

Symptoms Relieved

_____
_____
_____
_____
_____

Notes

_____
_____
_____
_____
_____
_____
_____

Effects	Strength
Peaceful	○ ○ ○ ○ ○
Sleepy	○ ○ ○ ○ ○
Pain Relief	○ ○ ○ ○ ○
Hungry	○ ○ ○ ○ ○
Uplifted	○ ○ ○ ○ ○
Creative	○ ○ ○ ○ ○

Ratings ☆ ☆ ☆ ☆ ☆

Strain

Grower _____   Date _____

Acquired _____ $ _____

| Indica | Hybrid | Sativa |

☐ Flower   ☐ Edible   ☐ Concentrate

Symptoms Relieved

_____
_____
_____
_____
_____

Sweet · Floral · Spicy · Herbal · Woodsy · Earthy · Sour · Fruity

Notes

_____
_____
_____
_____
_____
_____
_____

Effects	Strength
Peaceful	○ ○ ○ ○ ○
Sleepy	○ ○ ○ ○ ○
Pain Relief	○ ○ ○ ○ ○
Hungry	○ ○ ○ ○ ○
Uplifted	○ ○ ○ ○ ○
Creative	○ ○ ○ ○ ○

Ratings ☆ ☆ ☆ ☆ ☆

Strain

Grower _____ Date _____

Acquired _____ $ _____

| Indica | Hybrid | Sativa |

☐ Flower ☐ Edible ☐ Concentrate

Flavor wheel: Sweet, Floral, Spicy, Herbal, Woodsy, Earthy, Sour, Fruity

Symptoms Relieved

_____
_____
_____
_____

Notes

_____
_____
_____
_____
_____
_____

Effects	Strength
Peaceful	○ ○ ○ ○ ○
Sleepy	○ ○ ○ ○ ○
Pain Relief	○ ○ ○ ○ ○
Hungry	○ ○ ○ ○ ○
Uplifted	○ ○ ○ ○ ○
Creative	○ ○ ○ ○ ○

Ratings ☆ ☆ ☆ ☆ ☆

Strain

Grower _____ Date _____

Acquired _____ $ _____

| Indica | Hybrid | Sativa |

☐ Flower   ☐ Edible   ☐ Concentrate

Symptoms Relieved

_____
_____
_____
_____

Sweet · Fruity · Floral · Sour · Spicy · Earthy · Herbal · Woodsy

Notes

_____
_____
_____
_____
_____
_____

Effects	Strength
Peaceful	○ ○ ○ ○ ○
Sleepy	○ ○ ○ ○ ○
Pain Relief	○ ○ ○ ○ ○
Hungry	○ ○ ○ ○ ○
Uplifted	○ ○ ○ ○ ○
Creative	○ ○ ○ ○ ○

Ratings ☆ ☆ ☆ ☆ ☆

Strain

Grower _____ Date _____

Acquired _____ $ _____

| Indica | Hybrid | Sativa |

☐ Flower ☐ Edible ☐ Concentrate

Symptoms Relieved

_____
_____
_____
_____
_____

Sweet / Fruity / Floral / Sour / Spicy / Earthy / Woodsy / Herbal

Notes

_____
_____
_____
_____
_____
_____
_____

Effects	Strength
Peaceful	○ ○ ○ ○ ○
Sleepy	○ ○ ○ ○ ○
Pain Relief	○ ○ ○ ○ ○
Hungry	○ ○ ○ ○ ○
Uplifted	○ ○ ○ ○ ○
Creative	○ ○ ○ ○ ○

Ratings ☆ ☆ ☆ ☆ ☆

Strain

Grower: _____   Date: _____

Acquired: _____ $ _____

| Indica | Hybrid | Sativa |

☐ Flower ☐ Edible ☐ Concentrate

Symptoms Relieved

_____
_____
_____
_____

Sweet · Floral · Spicy · Herbal · Woodsy · Earthy · Sour · Fruity

Notes

_____
_____
_____
_____
_____

Effects	Strength
Peaceful	○ ○ ○ ○ ○
Sleepy	○ ○ ○ ○ ○
Pain Relief	○ ○ ○ ○ ○
Hungry	○ ○ ○ ○ ○
Uplifted	○ ○ ○ ○ ○
Creative	○ ○ ○ ○ ○

Ratings ☆ ☆ ☆ ☆ ☆

Strain

Grower _____ Date _____

Acquired _____ $ _____

Indica   Hybrid   Sativa

☐ Flower   ☐ Edible   ☐ Concentrate

Sweet
Fruity — Floral
Sour — Spicy
Earthy — Herbal
Woodsy

Symptoms Relieved

_____

_____

_____

_____

_____

Notes

_____

_____

_____

_____

_____

_____

Effects	Strength
Peaceful	○ ○ ○ ○ ○
Sleepy	○ ○ ○ ○ ○
Pain Relief	○ ○ ○ ○ ○
Hungry	○ ○ ○ ○ ○
Uplifted	○ ○ ○ ○ ○
Creative	○ ○ ○ ○ ○

Ratings ☆ ☆ ☆ ☆ ☆

Strain

Grower _____ Date _____

Acquired _____ $ _____

| Indica | Hybrid | Sativa |

☐ Flower   ☐ Edible   ☐ Concentrate

```
           Sweet
    Fruity       Floral

Sour                    Spicy

    Earthy       Herbal
           Woodsy
```

Symptoms Relieved

_____
_____
_____
_____

Notes

_____
_____
_____
_____
_____
_____

Effects	Strength
Peaceful	○ ○ ○ ○ ○
Sleepy	○ ○ ○ ○ ○
Pain Relief	○ ○ ○ ○ ○
Hungry	○ ○ ○ ○ ○
Uplifted	○ ○ ○ ○ ○
Creative	○ ○ ○ ○ ○

Ratings ☆ ☆ ☆ ☆ ☆

Strain

Grower _____ Date _____

Acquired _____ $ _____

Indica   Hybrid   Sativa

☐ Flower   ☐ Edible   ☐ Concentrate

Sweet
Fruity   Floral
Sour   Spicy
Earthy   Herbal
Woodsy

Symptoms Relieved

_____
_____
_____
_____

Notes

_____
_____
_____
_____
_____
_____

Effects	Strength
Peaceful	○ ○ ○ ○ ○
Sleepy	○ ○ ○ ○ ○
Pain Relief	○ ○ ○ ○ ○
Hungry	○ ○ ○ ○ ○
Uplifted	○ ○ ○ ○ ○
Creative	○ ○ ○ ○ ○

Ratings ☆ ☆ ☆ ☆ ☆

Strain

Grower _____ Date _____

Acquired _____ $ _____

| Indica | Hybrid | Sativa |

☐ Flower ☐ Edible ☐ Concentrate

Symptoms Relieved

_____
_____
_____
_____
_____

Sweet
Fruity   Floral
Sour   Spicy
Earthy   Herbal
Woodsy

Notes

_____
_____
_____
_____
_____
_____

Effects	Strength
Peaceful	○ ○ ○ ○ ○
Sleepy	○ ○ ○ ○ ○
Pain Relief	○ ○ ○ ○ ○
Hungry	○ ○ ○ ○ ○
Uplifted	○ ○ ○ ○ ○
Creative	○ ○ ○ ○ ○

Ratings ☆ ☆ ☆ ☆ ☆

Strain

Grower _____ Date _____

Acquired _____ $ _____

| Indica | Hybrid | Sativa |

☐ Flower ☐ Edible ☐ Concentrate

Sweet
Fruity   Floral
Sour   Spicy
Earthy   Herbal
Woodsy

Symptoms Relieved

_____
_____
_____
_____

Notes

_____
_____
_____
_____
_____
_____
_____

Effects	Strength
Peaceful	○ ○ ○ ○ ○
Sleepy	○ ○ ○ ○ ○
Pain Relief	○ ○ ○ ○ ○
Hungry	○ ○ ○ ○ ○
Uplifted	○ ○ ○ ○ ○
Creative	○ ○ ○ ○ ○

Ratings ☆ ☆ ☆ ☆ ☆

Strain

Grower _____ Date _____

Acquired _____ $ _____

| Indica | Hybrid | Sativa |

☐ Flower ☐ Edible ☐ Concentrate

Symptoms Relieved

_____
_____
_____
_____

Sweet · Floral · Spicy · Herbal · Woodsy · Earthy · Sour · Fruity

Notes

_____
_____
_____
_____
_____
_____

Effects	Strength
Peaceful	○ ○ ○ ○ ○
Sleepy	○ ○ ○ ○ ○
Pain Relief	○ ○ ○ ○ ○
Hungry	○ ○ ○ ○ ○
Uplifted	○ ○ ○ ○ ○
Creative	○ ○ ○ ○ ○

Ratings ☆ ☆ ☆ ☆ ☆

Strain

Grower _____ Date _____

Acquired _____ $ _____

| Indica | Hybrid | Sativa |

☐ Flower   ☐ Edible   ☐ Concentrate

Sweet · Fruity · Floral · Sour · Spicy · Earthy · Herbal · Woodsy

Symptoms Relieved

_____
_____
_____
_____
_____

Notes

_____
_____
_____
_____
_____
_____

Effects	Strength
Peaceful	○ ○ ○ ○ ○
Sleepy	○ ○ ○ ○ ○
Pain Relief	○ ○ ○ ○ ○
Hungry	○ ○ ○ ○ ○
Uplifted	○ ○ ○ ○ ○
Creative	○ ○ ○ ○ ○

Ratings ☆ ☆ ☆ ☆ ☆

Strain

Grower _____ Date _____

Acquired _____ $ _____

| Indica | Hybrid | Sativa |

☐ Flower ☐ Edible ☐ Concentrate

Symptoms Relieved

_____
_____
_____
_____

Sweet
Fruity
Floral
Sour
Spicy
Earthy
Herbal
Woodsy

Notes

_____
_____
_____
_____
_____
_____

Effects	Strength
Peaceful	○ ○ ○ ○ ○
Sleepy	○ ○ ○ ○ ○
Pain Relief	○ ○ ○ ○ ○
Hungry	○ ○ ○ ○ ○
Uplifted	○ ○ ○ ○ ○
Creative	○ ○ ○ ○ ○

Ratings ☆ ☆ ☆ ☆ ☆

Strain

Grower _____ Date _____

Acquired _____ $ _____

Indica　　　　Hybrid　　　　Sativa

☐ Flower　☐ Edible　☐ Concentrate

Sweet · Floral · Spicy · Herbal · Woodsy · Earthy · Sour · Fruity

Symptoms Relieved

_____
_____
_____
_____

Notes

_____
_____
_____
_____
_____
_____
_____

Effects	Strength
Peaceful	○ ○ ○ ○ ○
Sleepy	○ ○ ○ ○ ○
Pain Relief	○ ○ ○ ○ ○
Hungry	○ ○ ○ ○ ○
Uplifted	○ ○ ○ ○ ○
Creative	○ ○ ○ ○ ○

Ratings ☆ ☆ ☆ ☆ ☆

Strain

Grower _____ Date _____

Acquired _____ $ _____

| Indica | Hybrid | Sativa |

☐ Flower ☐ Edible ☐ Concentrate

Symptoms Relieved

_____
_____
_____
_____
_____

Sweet · Floral · Spicy · Herbal · Woodsy · Earthy · Sour · Fruity

Notes

_____
_____
_____
_____
_____
_____
_____

Effects	Strength
Peaceful	○ ○ ○ ○ ○
Sleepy	○ ○ ○ ○ ○
Pain Relief	○ ○ ○ ○ ○
Hungry	○ ○ ○ ○ ○
Uplifted	○ ○ ○ ○ ○
Creative	○ ○ ○ ○ ○

Ratings ☆ ☆ ☆ ☆ ☆

Strain

Grower _____ Date _____

Acquired _____ $ _____

| Indica | Hybrid | Sativa |

☐ Flower   ☐ Edible   ☐ Concentrate

Sweet
Fruity — Floral
Sour — Spicy
Earthy — Herbal
Woodsy

Symptoms Relieved

_____
_____
_____
_____

Notes

_____
_____
_____
_____
_____
_____
_____

Effects   **Strength**

Peaceful   ○ ○ ○ ○ ○
Sleepy   ○ ○ ○ ○ ○
Pain Relief ○ ○ ○ ○ ○
Hungry   ○ ○ ○ ○ ○
Uplifted   ○ ○ ○ ○ ○
Creative   ○ ○ ○ ○ ○

Ratings ☆ ☆ ☆ ☆ ☆

Strain

Grower _____ Date _____

Acquired _____ $ _____

| Indica | Hybrid | Sativa |

☐ Flower ☐ Edible ☐ Concentrate

Symptoms Relieved

_____
_____
_____
_____

Flavor wheel: Sweet, Floral, Spicy, Herbal, Woodsy, Earthy, Sour, Fruity

Notes

_____
_____
_____
_____
_____

Effects	Strength
Peaceful	○ ○ ○ ○ ○
Sleepy	○ ○ ○ ○ ○
Pain Relief	○ ○ ○ ○ ○
Hungry	○ ○ ○ ○ ○
Uplifted	○ ○ ○ ○ ○
Creative	○ ○ ○ ○ ○

Ratings ☆ ☆ ☆ ☆ ☆

Strain

Grower _____ Date _____

Acquired _____ $ _____

| Indica | Hybrid | Sativa |

☐ Flower   ☐ Edible   ☐ Concentrate

Symptoms Relieved

_____
_____
_____
_____
_____

Sweet / Floral / Spicy / Herbal / Woodsy / Earthy / Sour / Fruity

Notes

_____
_____
_____
_____
_____
_____
_____

Effects	Strength
Peaceful	○ ○ ○ ○ ○
Sleepy	○ ○ ○ ○ ○
Pain Relief	○ ○ ○ ○ ○
Hungry	○ ○ ○ ○ ○
Uplifted	○ ○ ○ ○ ○
Creative	○ ○ ○ ○ ○

Ratings ☆ ☆ ☆ ☆ ☆

Strain

Grower _____   Date _____

Acquired _____ $ _____

| Indica | Hybrid | Sativa |

☐ Flower   ☐ Edible   ☐ Concentrate

Symptoms Relieved
_____
_____
_____
_____
_____

Sweet
Fruity   Floral

Sour   Spicy

Earthy   Herbal
Woodsy

Notes
_____
_____
_____
_____
_____
_____
_____

Effects	Strength
Peaceful	○ ○ ○ ○ ○
Sleepy	○ ○ ○ ○ ○
Pain Relief	○ ○ ○ ○ ○
Hungry	○ ○ ○ ○ ○
Uplifted	○ ○ ○ ○ ○
Creative	○ ○ ○ ○ ○

Ratings ☆ ☆ ☆ ☆ ☆

Strain

Grower _____ Date _____

Acquired _____ $ _____

| Indica | Hybrid | Sativa |

☐ Flower   ☐ Edible   ☐ Concentrate

Symptoms Relieved

_____
_____
_____
_____

Sweet
Fruity   Floral
Sour   Spicy
Earthy   Herbal
Woodsy

Notes

_____
_____
_____
_____
_____
_____

Effects	Strength
Peaceful	○ ○ ○ ○ ○
Sleepy	○ ○ ○ ○ ○
Pain Relief	○ ○ ○ ○ ○
Hungry	○ ○ ○ ○ ○
Uplifted	○ ○ ○ ○ ○
Creative	○ ○ ○ ○ ○

Ratings ☆ ☆ ☆ ☆ ☆

Strain

Grower _____ Date _____

Acquired _____ $ _____

| Indica | Hybrid | Sativa |

☐ Flower   ☐ Edible   ☐ Concentrate

Symptoms Relieved

_____
_____
_____
_____

Sweet
Fruity — Floral
Sour — Spicy
Earthy — Herbal
Woodsy

Notes

_____
_____
_____
_____
_____
_____
_____

Effects	Strength
Peaceful	○ ○ ○ ○ ○
Sleepy	○ ○ ○ ○ ○
Pain Relief	○ ○ ○ ○ ○
Hungry	○ ○ ○ ○ ○
Uplifted	○ ○ ○ ○ ○
Creative	○ ○ ○ ○ ○

Ratings ☆ ☆ ☆ ☆ ☆

Strain

Grower _____ Date _____

Acquired _____ $ _____

Indica   Hybrid   Sativa

☐ Flower   ☐ Edible   ☐ Concentrate

Symptoms Relieved

_____
_____
_____
_____

Sweet / Fruity / Floral / Sour / Spicy / Earthy / Herbal / Woodsy

Notes

_____
_____
_____
_____
_____
_____

Effects	Strength
Peaceful	○ ○ ○ ○ ○
Sleepy	○ ○ ○ ○ ○
Pain Relief	○ ○ ○ ○ ○
Hungry	○ ○ ○ ○ ○
Uplifted	○ ○ ○ ○ ○
Creative	○ ○ ○ ○ ○

Ratings ☆ ☆ ☆ ☆ ☆

Strain

Grower _____ Date _____

Acquired _____ $ _____

| Indica | Hybrid | Sativa |

☐ Flower ☐ Edible ☐ Concentrate

Symptoms Relieved

_____
_____
_____
_____
_____

Sweet · Floral · Spicy · Herbal · Woodsy · Earthy · Sour · Fruity

Notes

_____
_____
_____
_____
_____
_____

Effects	Strength
Peaceful	○ ○ ○ ○ ○
Sleepy	○ ○ ○ ○ ○
Pain Relief	○ ○ ○ ○ ○
Hungry	○ ○ ○ ○ ○
Uplifted	○ ○ ○ ○ ○
Creative	○ ○ ○ ○ ○

Ratings ☆ ☆ ☆ ☆ ☆

Strain

Grower _____   Date _____

Acquired _____ $ _____

Indica	Hybrid	Sativa

☐ Flower   ☐ Edible   ☐ Concentrate

Sweet
Fruity   Floral
Sour   Spicy
Earthy   Herbal
Woodsy

Symptoms Relieved

_____
_____
_____
_____
_____

Notes

_____
_____
_____
_____
_____
_____
_____

Effects	Strength
Peaceful	○ ○ ○ ○ ○
Sleepy	○ ○ ○ ○ ○
Pain Relief	○ ○ ○ ○ ○
Hungry	○ ○ ○ ○ ○
Uplifted	○ ○ ○ ○ ○
Creative	○ ○ ○ ○ ○

Ratings ☆ ☆ ☆ ☆ ☆

Strain

Grower _____ Date _____

Acquired _____ $ _____

| Indica | Hybrid | Sativa |

☐ Flower ☐ Edible ☐ Concentrate

```
              Sweet
      Fruity        Floral

  Sour                    Spicy

      Earthy        Herbal
              Woodsy
```

Symptoms Relieved

_____
_____
_____
_____
_____

Notes

_____
_____
_____
_____
_____
_____
_____

Effects	Strength
Peaceful	○ ○ ○ ○ ○
Sleepy	○ ○ ○ ○ ○
Pain Relief	○ ○ ○ ○ ○
Hungry	○ ○ ○ ○ ○
Uplifted	○ ○ ○ ○ ○
Creative	○ ○ ○ ○ ○

Ratings ☆ ☆ ☆ ☆ ☆

Strain

Grower _____ Date _____

Acquired _____ $ _____

Indica   Hybrid   Sativa

☐ Flower   ☐ Edible   ☐ Concentrate

Sweet, Fruity, Floral, Sour, Spicy, Earthy, Woodsy, Herbal

Symptoms Relieved

_____
_____
_____
_____

Notes

_____
_____
_____
_____
_____
_____

Effects	Strength
Peaceful	○ ○ ○ ○ ○
Sleepy	○ ○ ○ ○ ○
Pain Relief	○ ○ ○ ○ ○
Hungry	○ ○ ○ ○ ○
Uplifted	○ ○ ○ ○ ○
Creative	○ ○ ○ ○ ○

Ratings ☆ ☆ ☆ ☆ ☆

Strain

Grower _____   Date _____

Acquired _____ $ _____

| Indica | Hybrid | Sativa |

☐ Flower ☐ Edible ☐ Concentrate

Symptoms Relieved
_____
_____
_____
_____
_____

Flavor wheel: Sweet, Floral, Spicy, Herbal, Woodsy, Earthy, Sour, Fruity

Notes
_____
_____
_____
_____
_____
_____
_____

Effects	Strength
Peaceful	○ ○ ○ ○ ○
Sleepy	○ ○ ○ ○ ○
Pain Relief	○ ○ ○ ○ ○
Hungry	○ ○ ○ ○ ○
Uplifted	○ ○ ○ ○ ○
Creative	○ ○ ○ ○ ○

Ratings ☆ ☆ ☆ ☆ ☆

Strain

Grower _____   Date _____

Acquired _____ $ _____

| Indica | Hybrid | Sativa |

☐ Flower ☐ Edible ☐ Concentrate

Sweet · Fruity · Floral · Sour · Spicy · Earthy · Herbal · Woodsy

Symptoms Relieved

_____
_____
_____
_____

Notes

_____
_____
_____
_____
_____
_____

Effects	Strength
Peaceful	○ ○ ○ ○ ○
Sleepy	○ ○ ○ ○ ○
Pain Relief	○ ○ ○ ○ ○
Hungry	○ ○ ○ ○ ○
Uplifted	○ ○ ○ ○ ○
Creative	○ ○ ○ ○ ○

Ratings ☆ ☆ ☆ ☆ ☆

Strain

Grower _____ Date _____

Acquired _____ $ _____

| Indica | Hybrid | Sativa |

☐ Flower ☐ Edible ☐ Concentrate

Sweet
Fruity   Floral
Sour   Spicy
Earthy   Herbal
Woodsy

Symptoms Relieved

_____
_____
_____
_____
_____

Notes

_____
_____
_____
_____
_____
_____

Effects	Strength
Peaceful	○ ○ ○ ○ ○
Sleepy	○ ○ ○ ○ ○
Pain Relief	○ ○ ○ ○ ○
Hungry	○ ○ ○ ○ ○
Uplifted	○ ○ ○ ○ ○
Creative	○ ○ ○ ○ ○

Ratings ☆ ☆ ☆ ☆ ☆

Strain

Grower _____ Date _____

Acquired _____ $ _____

| Indica | Hybrid | Sativa |

☐ Flower   ☐ Edible   ☐ Concentrate

Symptoms Relieved

_____
_____
_____
_____

Sweet / Fruity / Floral / Sour / Spicy / Earthy / Woodsy / Herbal

Notes

_____
_____
_____
_____
_____
_____

Effects	Strength
Peaceful	○ ○ ○ ○ ○
Sleepy	○ ○ ○ ○ ○
Pain Relief	○ ○ ○ ○ ○
Hungry	○ ○ ○ ○ ○
Uplifted	○ ○ ○ ○ ○
Creative	○ ○ ○ ○ ○

Ratings ☆ ☆ ☆ ☆ ☆

Strain

Grower _____ Date _____

Acquired _____ $ _____

| Indica | Hybrid | Sativa |

☐ Flower ☐ Edible ☐ Concentrate

Symptoms Relieved

_____
_____
_____
_____
_____

Sweet
Fruity
Floral
Sour
Spicy
Earthy
Herbal
Woodsy

Notes

_____
_____
_____
_____
_____
_____
_____

Effects	Strength
Peaceful	○ ○ ○ ○ ○
Sleepy	○ ○ ○ ○ ○
Pain Relief	○ ○ ○ ○ ○
Hungry	○ ○ ○ ○ ○
Uplifted	○ ○ ○ ○ ○
Creative	○ ○ ○ ○ ○

Ratings ☆ ☆ ☆ ☆ ☆

Strain

Grower _____ Date _____

Acquired _____ $ _____

Indica   Hybrid   Sativa

☐ Flower   ☐ Edible   ☐ Concentrate

Sweet
Fruity   Floral
Sour   Spicy
Earthy   Herbal
Woodsy

Symptoms Relieved

_____
_____
_____
_____

Notes

_____
_____
_____
_____
_____
_____
_____

Effects	Strength
Peaceful	○ ○ ○ ○ ○
Sleepy	○ ○ ○ ○ ○
Pain Relief	○ ○ ○ ○ ○
Hungry	○ ○ ○ ○ ○
Uplifted	○ ○ ○ ○ ○
Creative	○ ○ ○ ○ ○

Ratings ☆ ☆ ☆ ☆ ☆

Strain

Grower _____   Date _____

Acquired _____ $ _____

Indica	Hybrid	Sativa

☐ Flower   ☐ Edible   ☐ Concentrate

Symptoms Relieved

_____
_____
_____
_____
_____

Sweet • Floral • Spicy • Herbal • Woodsy • Earthy • Sour • Fruity

Notes

_____
_____
_____
_____
_____
_____
_____

Effects	Strength
Peaceful	○ ○ ○ ○ ○
Sleepy	○ ○ ○ ○ ○
Pain Relief	○ ○ ○ ○ ○
Hungry	○ ○ ○ ○ ○
Uplifted	○ ○ ○ ○ ○
Creative	○ ○ ○ ○ ○

Ratings ☆ ☆ ☆ ☆ ☆

Strain

Grower _____   Date _____

Acquired _____ $ _____

| Indica | Hybrid | Sativa |

☐ Flower   ☐ Edible   ☐ Concentrate

Symptoms Relieved

_____
_____
_____
_____

Flavor wheel: Sweet, Floral, Spicy, Herbal, Woodsy, Earthy, Sour, Fruity

Notes

_____
_____
_____
_____
_____
_____

Effects	Strength
Peaceful	○ ○ ○ ○ ○
Sleepy	○ ○ ○ ○ ○
Pain Relief	○ ○ ○ ○ ○
Hungry	○ ○ ○ ○ ○
Uplifted	○ ○ ○ ○ ○
Creative	○ ○ ○ ○ ○

Ratings ☆ ☆ ☆ ☆ ☆

Strain

Grower _____ Date _____

Acquired _____ $ _____

| Indica | Hybrid | Sativa |

☐ Flower   ☐ Edible   ☐ Concentrate

Symptoms Relieved

_____

_____

_____

_____

Sweet · Floral · Spicy · Herbal · Woodsy · Earthy · Sour · Fruity

Notes

_____

_____

_____

_____

_____

Effects	Strength
Peaceful	○ ○ ○ ○ ○
Sleepy	○ ○ ○ ○ ○
Pain Relief	○ ○ ○ ○ ○
Hungry	○ ○ ○ ○ ○
Uplifted	○ ○ ○ ○ ○
Creative	○ ○ ○ ○ ○

Ratings ☆ ☆ ☆ ☆ ☆

Strain

Grower _____ Date _____

Acquired _____ $ _____

| Indica | Hybrid | Sativa |

☐ Flower   ☐ Edible   ☐ Concentrate

Symptoms Relieved

_____
_____
_____
_____
_____

Sweet · Floral · Spicy · Herbal · Woodsy · Earthy · Sour · Fruity

Notes

_____
_____
_____
_____
_____
_____
_____

Effects	Strength
Peaceful	○ ○ ○ ○ ○
Sleepy	○ ○ ○ ○ ○
Pain Relief	○ ○ ○ ○ ○
Hungry	○ ○ ○ ○ ○
Uplifted	○ ○ ○ ○ ○
Creative	○ ○ ○ ○ ○

Ratings ☆ ☆ ☆ ☆ ☆

Strain

Grower _____ Date _____

Acquired _____ $ _____

| Indica | Hybrid | Sativa |

☐ Flower   ☐ Edible   ☐ Concentrate

Sweet
Fruity   Floral
Sour   Spicy
Earthy   Herbal
Woodsy

Symptoms Relieved

_____
_____
_____
_____

Notes

_____
_____
_____
_____
_____
_____

Effects	**Strength**
Peaceful	○ ○ ○ ○ ○
Sleepy	○ ○ ○ ○ ○
Pain Relief	○ ○ ○ ○ ○
Hungry	○ ○ ○ ○ ○
Uplifted	○ ○ ○ ○ ○
Creative	○ ○ ○ ○ ○

Ratings ☆ ☆ ☆ ☆ ☆

Strain

Grower _____   Date _____

Acquired _____ $ _____

| Indica | Hybrid | Sativa |

☐ Flower   ☐ Edible   ☐ Concentrate

Symptoms Relieved
_____
_____
_____
_____

Notes
_____
_____
_____
_____
_____
_____

Flavor wheel: Sweet, Floral, Spicy, Herbal, Woodsy, Earthy, Sour, Fruity

Effects	Strength
Peaceful	○ ○ ○ ○ ○
Sleepy	○ ○ ○ ○ ○
Pain Relief	○ ○ ○ ○ ○
Hungry	○ ○ ○ ○ ○
Uplifted	○ ○ ○ ○ ○
Creative	○ ○ ○ ○ ○

Ratings ☆ ☆ ☆ ☆ ☆

Strain

Grower _____ Date _____

Acquired _____ $ _____

| Indica | Hybrid | Sativa |

☐ Flower ☐ Edible ☐ Concentrate

Symptoms Relieved

_____
_____
_____
_____

Sweet · Floral · Spicy · Herbal · Woodsy · Earthy · Sour · Fruity

Notes

_____
_____
_____
_____
_____
_____

Effects	Strength
Peaceful	○ ○ ○ ○ ○
Sleepy	○ ○ ○ ○ ○
Pain Relief	○ ○ ○ ○ ○
Hungry	○ ○ ○ ○ ○
Uplifted	○ ○ ○ ○ ○
Creative	○ ○ ○ ○ ○

Ratings ☆ ☆ ☆ ☆ ☆

Strain

Grower _____ Date _____

Acquired _____ $ _____

| Indica | Hybrid | Sativa |

☐ Flower   ☐ Edible   ☐ Concentrate

Symptoms Relieved

_____
_____
_____
_____

Sweet · Fruity · Floral · Sour · Spicy · Earthy · Herbal · Woodsy

Notes

_____
_____
_____
_____
_____
_____

Effects	Strength
Peaceful	○ ○ ○ ○ ○
Sleepy	○ ○ ○ ○ ○
Pain Relief	○ ○ ○ ○ ○
Hungry	○ ○ ○ ○ ○
Uplifted	○ ○ ○ ○ ○
Creative	○ ○ ○ ○ ○

Ratings ☆ ☆ ☆ ☆ ☆

Strain

Grower _____ Date _____

Acquired _____ $ _____

| Indica | Hybrid | Sativa |

☐ Flower ☐ Edible ☐ Concentrate

Symptoms Relieved

_____
_____
_____
_____

Sweet · Floral · Spicy · Herbal · Woodsy · Earthy · Sour · Fruity

Notes

_____
_____
_____
_____
_____
_____

Effects	Strength
Peaceful	○ ○ ○ ○ ○
Sleepy	○ ○ ○ ○ ○
Pain Relief	○ ○ ○ ○ ○
Hungry	○ ○ ○ ○ ○
Uplifted	○ ○ ○ ○ ○
Creative	○ ○ ○ ○ ○

Ratings ☆ ☆ ☆ ☆ ☆

Strain

Grower _____   Date _____

Acquired _____ $ _____

| Indica | Hybrid | Sativa |

☐ Flower   ☐ Edible   ☐ Concentrate

Symptoms Relieved

_____
_____
_____
_____
_____

Sweet · Floral · Spicy · Herbal · Woodsy · Earthy · Sour · Fruity

Notes

_____
_____
_____
_____
_____
_____
_____

Effects	Strength
Peaceful	○ ○ ○ ○ ○
Sleepy	○ ○ ○ ○ ○
Pain Relief	○ ○ ○ ○ ○
Hungry	○ ○ ○ ○ ○
Uplifted	○ ○ ○ ○ ○
Creative	○ ○ ○ ○ ○

Ratings ☆ ☆ ☆ ☆ ☆

Strain

Grower _____ Date _____

Acquired _____ $ _____

| Indica | Hybrid | Sativa |

☐ Flower ☐ Edible ☐ Concentrate

Symptoms Relieved

_____
_____
_____
_____
_____

Sweet
Fruity   Floral
Sour   Spicy
Earthy   Herbal
Woodsy

Notes

_____
_____
_____
_____
_____
_____
_____

Effects	Strength
Peaceful	○ ○ ○ ○ ○
Sleepy	○ ○ ○ ○ ○
Pain Relief	○ ○ ○ ○ ○
Hungry	○ ○ ○ ○ ○
Uplifted	○ ○ ○ ○ ○
Creative	○ ○ ○ ○ ○

Ratings ☆ ☆ ☆ ☆ ☆

Strain

Grower _____ Date _____

Acquired _____ $ _____

| Indica | Hybrid | Sativa |

☐ Flower   ☐ Edible   ☐ Concentrate

Symptoms Relieved

_____
_____
_____
_____

Sweet · Floral · Spicy · Herbal · Woodsy · Earthy · Sour · Fruity

Notes

_____
_____
_____
_____
_____
_____

Effects	Strength
Peaceful	○ ○ ○ ○ ○
Sleepy	○ ○ ○ ○ ○
Pain Relief	○ ○ ○ ○ ○
Hungry	○ ○ ○ ○ ○
Uplifted	○ ○ ○ ○ ○
Creative	○ ○ ○ ○ ○

Ratings ☆ ☆ ☆ ☆

Strain

Grower _____ Date _____

Acquired _____ $ _____

| Indica | Hybrid | Sativa |

☐ Flower ☐ Edible ☐ Concentrate

Sweet
Fruity — Floral
Sour — Spicy
Earthy — Herbal
Woodsy

Symptoms Relieved
_____
_____
_____
_____

Notes
_____
_____
_____
_____
_____
_____

Effects	Strength
Peaceful	○ ○ ○ ○ ○
Sleepy	○ ○ ○ ○ ○
Pain Relief	○ ○ ○ ○ ○
Hungry	○ ○ ○ ○ ○
Uplifted	○ ○ ○ ○ ○
Creative	○ ○ ○ ○ ○

Ratings ☆ ☆ ☆ ☆ ☆

Strain

Grower _____ Date _____

Acquired _____ $ _____

| Indica | Hybrid | Sativa |

☐ Flower ☐ Edible ☐ Concentrate

Sweet
Fruity   Floral

Sour   Spicy

Earthy   Herbal
Woodsy

Symptoms Relieved

_____
_____
_____
_____

Notes

_____
_____
_____
_____
_____
_____
_____

Effects	Strength
Peaceful	○ ○ ○ ○ ○
Sleepy	○ ○ ○ ○ ○
Pain Relief	○ ○ ○ ○ ○
Hungry	○ ○ ○ ○ ○
Uplifted	○ ○ ○ ○ ○
Creative	○ ○ ○ ○ ○

Ratings ☆ ☆ ☆ ☆ ☆

Strain

Grower _____ Date _____

Acquired _____ $ _____

| Indica | Hybrid | Sativa |

☐ Flower ☐ Edible ☐ Concentrate

Sweet
Fruity — Floral
Sour — Spicy
Earthy — Herbal
Woodsy

Symptoms Relieved

_____
_____
_____
_____

Notes

_____
_____
_____
_____

Effects	Strength
Peaceful	○ ○ ○ ○ ○
Sleepy	○ ○ ○ ○ ○
Pain Relief	○ ○ ○ ○ ○
Hungry	○ ○ ○ ○ ○
Uplifted	○ ○ ○ ○ ○
Creative	○ ○ ○ ○ ○

Ratings ☆ ☆ ☆ ☆ ☆

Strain

Grower _____ Date _____

Acquired _____ $ _____

Indica	Hybrid	Sativa

☐ Flower ☐ Edible ☐ Concentrate

Symptoms Relieved

_____
_____
_____
_____
_____

Sweet · Floral · Spicy · Herbal · Woodsy · Earthy · Sour · Fruity

Notes

_____
_____
_____
_____
_____
_____

Effects	Strength
Peaceful	○ ○ ○ ○ ○
Sleepy	○ ○ ○ ○ ○
Pain Relief	○ ○ ○ ○ ○
Hungry	○ ○ ○ ○ ○
Uplifted	○ ○ ○ ○ ○
Creative	○ ○ ○ ○ ○

Ratings ☆ ☆ ☆ ☆ ☆

Strain

Grower _____   Date _____

Acquired _____ $ _____

| Indica | Hybrid | Sativa |

☐ Flower ☐ Edible ☐ Concentrate

                Sweet
    Fruity   Floral

Symptoms Relieved

Sour   Spicy

_____

_____

_____

_____

    Earthy   Herbal
              Woodsy

Effects	**Strength**
Peaceful	○ ○ ○ ○ ○
Sleepy	○ ○ ○ ○ ○
Pain Relief	○ ○ ○ ○ ○
Hungry	○ ○ ○ ○ ○
Uplifted	○ ○ ○ ○ ○
Creative	○ ○ ○ ○ ○

Notes

_____

_____

_____

_____

_____

_____

_____

Ratings ☆ ☆ ☆ ☆ ☆

Strain

Grower _____ Date _____

Acquired _____ $ _____

Indica　　　Hybrid　　　Sativa

☐ Flower　☐ Edible　☐ Concentrate

Symptoms Relieved

_____
_____
_____
_____

Sweet / Floral / Spicy / Herbal / Woodsy / Earthy / Sour / Fruity

Notes

_____
_____
_____
_____
_____
_____

Effects	Strength
Peaceful	○ ○ ○ ○ ○
Sleepy	○ ○ ○ ○ ○
Pain Relief	○ ○ ○ ○ ○
Hungry	○ ○ ○ ○ ○
Uplifted	○ ○ ○ ○ ○
Creative	○ ○ ○ ○ ○

Ratings ☆ ☆ ☆ ☆ ☆

Strain

Grower _____   Date _____

Acquired _____ $ _____

| Indica | Hybrid | Sativa |

☐ Flower ☐ Edible ☐ Concentrate

Symptoms Relieved
_____
_____
_____
_____

Sweet · Floral · Spicy · Herbal · Woodsy · Earthy · Sour · Fruity

Notes
_____
_____
_____
_____
_____

Effects	Strength
Peaceful	○ ○ ○ ○ ○
Sleepy	○ ○ ○ ○ ○
Pain Relief	○ ○ ○ ○ ○
Hungry	○ ○ ○ ○ ○
Uplifted	○ ○ ○ ○ ○
Creative	○ ○ ○ ○ ○

Ratings ☆ ☆ ☆ ☆ ☆

Strain

Grower _____ Date _____

Acquired _____ $ _____

| Indica | Hybrid | Sativa |

☐ Flower ☐ Edible ☐ Concentrate

Sweet
Fruity   Floral
Sour   Spicy
Earthy   Herbal
Woodsy

Symptoms Relieved

_____
_____
_____
_____

Notes

_____
_____
_____
_____
_____
_____

Effects	**Strength**
Peaceful	○ ○ ○ ○ ○
Sleepy	○ ○ ○ ○ ○
Pain Relief	○ ○ ○ ○ ○
Hungry	○ ○ ○ ○ ○
Uplifted	○ ○ ○ ○ ○
Creative	○ ○ ○ ○ ○

Ratings ☆ ☆ ☆ ☆ ☆

Strain

Grower: _____ Date: _____

Acquired: _____ $ _____

| Indica | Hybrid | Sativa |

☐ Flower ☐ Edible ☐ Concentrate

Aroma wheel: Sweet, Floral, Spicy, Herbal, Woodsy, Earthy, Sour, Fruity

Symptoms Relieved

_____
_____
_____
_____

Notes

_____
_____
_____
_____
_____
_____

Effects	Strength
Peaceful	○ ○ ○ ○ ○
Sleepy	○ ○ ○ ○ ○
Pain Relief	○ ○ ○ ○ ○
Hungry	○ ○ ○ ○ ○
Uplifted	○ ○ ○ ○ ○
Creative	○ ○ ○ ○ ○

Ratings ☆ ☆ ☆ ☆ ☆

Strain

Grower: _____ Date: _____

Acquired: _____ $ _____

Indica　　　　　Hybrid　　　　　Sativa

☐ Flower　　☐ Edible　　☐ Concentrate

Symptoms Relieved

_____
_____
_____
_____
_____

Notes

_____
_____
_____
_____
_____
_____

Sweet · Floral · Spicy · Herbal · Woodsy · Earthy · Sour · Fruity

Effects	Strength
Peaceful	○ ○ ○ ○ ○
Sleepy	○ ○ ○ ○ ○
Pain Relief	○ ○ ○ ○ ○
Hungry	○ ○ ○ ○ ○
Uplifted	○ ○ ○ ○ ○
Creative	○ ○ ○ ○ ○

Ratings ☆ ☆ ☆ ☆ ☆

Strain

Grower _____ Date _____

Acquired _____ $ _____

| Indica | Hybrid | Sativa |

☐ Flower ☐ Edible ☐ Concentrate

Symptoms Relieved

_____
_____
_____
_____
_____

Sweet
Fruity — Floral
Sour — Spicy
Earthy — Herbal
Woodsy

Notes

_____
_____
_____
_____
_____
_____

Effects	Strength
Peaceful	○ ○ ○ ○ ○
Sleepy	○ ○ ○ ○ ○
Pain Relief	○ ○ ○ ○ ○
Hungry	○ ○ ○ ○ ○
Uplifted	○ ○ ○ ○ ○
Creative	○ ○ ○ ○ ○

Ratings ☆ ☆ ☆ ☆ ☆

Strain

Grower _____ Date _____

Acquired _____ $ _____

| Indica | Hybrid | Sativa |

☐ Flower   ☐ Edible   ☐ Concentrate

Sweet
Fruity   Floral
Sour   Spicy
Earthy   Herbal
Woodsy

Symptoms Relieved

_____
_____
_____
_____

Notes

_____
_____
_____
_____
_____
_____

Effects	Strength
Peaceful	○ ○ ○ ○ ○
Sleepy	○ ○ ○ ○ ○
Pain Relief	○ ○ ○ ○ ○
Hungry	○ ○ ○ ○ ○
Uplifted	○ ○ ○ ○ ○
Creative	○ ○ ○ ○ ○

Ratings ☆ ☆ ☆ ☆ ☆

Strain

Grower _____ Date _____

Acquired _____ $ _____

| Indica | Hybrid | Sativa |

☐ Flower ☐ Edible ☐ Concentrate

Symptoms Relieved

_____
_____
_____
_____

Sweet
Fruity — Floral
Sour — Spicy
Earthy — Herbal
Woodsy

Notes

_____
_____
_____
_____
_____
_____

Effects	Strength
Peaceful	○ ○ ○ ○ ○
Sleepy	○ ○ ○ ○ ○
Pain Relief	○ ○ ○ ○ ○
Hungry	○ ○ ○ ○ ○
Uplifted	○ ○ ○ ○ ○
Creative	○ ○ ○ ○ ○

Ratings ☆ ☆ ☆ ☆ ☆

Strain

Grower _____ Date _____

Acquired _____ $ _____

| Indica | Hybrid | Sativa |

☐ Flower ☐ Edible ☐ Concentrate

Symptoms Relieved

_____
_____
_____
_____

Sweet · Floral · Spicy · Herbal · Woodsy · Earthy · Sour · Fruity

Notes

_____
_____
_____
_____
_____
_____

Effects	Strength
Peaceful	○ ○ ○ ○ ○
Sleepy	○ ○ ○ ○ ○
Pain Relief	○ ○ ○ ○ ○
Hungry	○ ○ ○ ○ ○
Uplifted	○ ○ ○ ○ ○
Creative	○ ○ ○ ○ ○

Ratings ☆ ☆ ☆ ☆ ☆

Strain

Grower _____ Date _____

Acquired _____ $ _____

| Indica | Hybrid | Sativa |

☐ Flower ☐ Edible ☐ Concentrate

Symptoms Relieved

_____
_____
_____
_____

Sweet / Floral / Spicy / Herbal / Woodsy / Earthy / Sour / Fruity

Notes

_____
_____
_____
_____
_____

Effects	Strength
Peaceful	○ ○ ○ ○ ○
Sleepy	○ ○ ○ ○ ○
Pain Relief	○ ○ ○ ○ ○
Hungry	○ ○ ○ ○ ○
Uplifted	○ ○ ○ ○ ○
Creative	○ ○ ○ ○ ○

Ratings ☆ ☆ ☆ ☆ ☆

Strain

Grower _____ Date _____

Acquired _____ $ _____

Indica Hybrid Sativa

☐ Flower ☐ Edible ☐ Concentrate

Sweet
Fruity Floral
Sour Spicy
Earthy Herbal
Woodsy

Symptoms Relieved

_____
_____
_____
_____

Notes

_____
_____
_____
_____
_____
_____

Effects	Strength
Peaceful	○ ○ ○ ○ ○
Sleepy	○ ○ ○ ○ ○
Pain Relief	○ ○ ○ ○ ○
Hungry	○ ○ ○ ○ ○
Uplifted	○ ○ ○ ○ ○
Creative	○ ○ ○ ○ ○

Ratings ☆ ☆ ☆ ☆ ☆

Strain

Grower _____ Date _____

Acquired _____ $ _____

| Indica | Hybrid | Sativa |

☐ Flower ☐ Edible ☐ Concentrate

Symptoms Relieved

_____
_____
_____
_____
_____

Sweet · Fruity · Floral · Sour · Spicy · Earthy · Herbal · Woodsy

Notes

_____
_____
_____
_____
_____
_____
_____

Effects	Strength
Peaceful	○ ○ ○ ○ ○
Sleepy	○ ○ ○ ○ ○
Pain Relief	○ ○ ○ ○ ○
Hungry	○ ○ ○ ○ ○
Uplifted	○ ○ ○ ○ ○
Creative	○ ○ ○ ○ ○

Ratings ☆ ☆ ☆ ☆ ☆

Strain

Grower _____ Date _____

Acquired _____ $ _____

| Indica | Hybrid | Sativa |

☐ Flower ☐ Edible ☐ Concentrate

Sweet
Fruity   Floral

Symptoms Relieved

Sour   Spicy

_____

_____

_____

_____

Earthy   Herbal
Woodsy

| Effects | Strength |

Notes

Peaceful ○ ○ ○ ○ ○

Sleepy ○ ○ ○ ○ ○

_____

Pain Relief ○ ○ ○ ○ ○

_____

Hungry ○ ○ ○ ○ ○

_____

Uplifted ○ ○ ○ ○ ○

_____

Creative ○ ○ ○ ○ ○

_____

Ratings ☆ ☆ ☆ ☆ ☆

Strain

Grower _____ Date _____

Acquired _____ $ _____

| Indica | Hybrid | Sativa |

☐ Flower ☐ Edible ☐ Concentrate

Symptoms Relieved

_____
_____
_____
_____

Flavor wheel: Sweet, Floral, Spicy, Herbal, Woodsy, Earthy, Sour, Fruity

Notes

_____
_____
_____
_____
_____
_____

Effects	Strength
Peaceful	○ ○ ○ ○ ○
Sleepy	○ ○ ○ ○ ○
Pain Relief	○ ○ ○ ○ ○
Hungry	○ ○ ○ ○ ○
Uplifted	○ ○ ○ ○ ○
Creative	○ ○ ○ ○ ○

Ratings ☆ ☆ ☆ ☆ ☆

Strain

Grower _____ Date _____

Acquired _____ $ _____

| Indica | Hybrid | Sativa |

☐ Flower ☐ Edible ☐ Concentrate

Sweet / Fruity / Floral / Sour / Spicy / Earthy / Herbal / Woodsy

Symptoms Relieved

_____
_____
_____
_____

Notes

_____
_____
_____
_____
_____
_____

Effects	Strength
Peaceful	○ ○ ○ ○ ○
Sleepy	○ ○ ○ ○ ○
Pain Relief	○ ○ ○ ○ ○
Hungry	○ ○ ○ ○ ○
Uplifted	○ ○ ○ ○ ○
Creative	○ ○ ○ ○ ○

Ratings ☆ ☆ ☆ ☆ ☆

Strain

Grower _____ Date _____

Acquired _____ $ _____

| Indica | Hybrid | Sativa |

☐ Flower ☐ Edible ☐ Concentrate

Symptoms Relieved

_____

_____

_____

_____

Sweet · Floral · Spicy · Herbal · Woodsy · Earthy · Sour · Fruity

Notes

_____

_____

_____

_____

_____

_____

Effects	Strength
Peaceful	○ ○ ○ ○ ○
Sleepy	○ ○ ○ ○ ○
Pain Relief	○ ○ ○ ○ ○
Hungry	○ ○ ○ ○ ○
Uplifted	○ ○ ○ ○ ○
Creative	○ ○ ○ ○ ○

Ratings ☆ ☆ ☆ ☆ ☆

Strain

Grower _____ Date _____

Acquired _____ $ _____

| Indica | Hybrid | Sativa |

☐ Flower ☐ Edible ☐ Concentrate

Sweet
Fruity — Floral
Sour — Spicy
Earthy — Herbal
Woodsy

Symptoms Relieved

_____
_____
_____
_____

Notes

_____
_____
_____
_____
_____
_____

Effects	Strength
Peaceful	○ ○ ○ ○ ○
Sleepy	○ ○ ○ ○ ○
Pain Relief	○ ○ ○ ○ ○
Hungry	○ ○ ○ ○ ○
Uplifted	○ ○ ○ ○ ○
Creative	○ ○ ○ ○ ○

Ratings ☆ ☆ ☆ ☆ ☆

Strain

Grower _____ Date _____

Acquired _____ $ _____

| Indica | Hybrid | Sativa |

☐ Flower   ☐ Edible   ☐ Concentrate

Sweet
Fruity   Floral
Sour   Spicy
Earthy   Herbal
Woodsy

Symptoms Relieved

_____
_____
_____
_____
_____

Notes

_____
_____
_____
_____
_____
_____
_____

Effects	Strength
Peaceful	○ ○ ○ ○ ○
Sleepy	○ ○ ○ ○ ○
Pain Relief	○ ○ ○ ○ ○
Hungry	○ ○ ○ ○ ○
Uplifted	○ ○ ○ ○ ○
Creative	○ ○ ○ ○ ○

Ratings ☆ ☆ ☆ ☆ ☆

Enjoy this book?

Why not check out our other titles on Amazon?

We also have a range of complimentary items available on our website

www.inspirational.media

Many thanks for your purchase!

© *Inspirational Media Publishing 2019*

Made in the USA
Coppell, TX
07 May 2024